your pregnancy™

Quick Guide

Fitness and Exercise

your
pregnancy™
Quick Guide

Fitness and Exercise

*What You Need to Know about Staying
in Shape during Your Pregnancy*

Glade B. Curtis, M.D., M.P.H., OB/GYN
Judith Schuler, M.S.

Da Capo
∞
LIFE
LONG

A Member of the Perseus Books Group

Text design by Brent Wilcox
Illustrations by Sara Mintz Zwicker
Set in 11.5 point Minion by the Perseus Books Group

Library of Congress Cataloging-in-Publication Data

Curtis, Glade B.
  Your pregnancy quick guide to fitness and exercise : what you need to know about staying in shape during your pregnancy / Glade B. Curtis and Judith Schuler.
    p.   cm.
  Includes index.
  ISBN 0-7382-0952-X (pbk. : alk. paper)
  1. Exercise for pregnant women.   2. Pregnant women—Health and hygiene.   I. Schuler, Judith.   II. Title.
RG558.7.C87 2004
618.2'44—dc22

                                                                                    2004010656

First Da Capo Press printing 2004

Published by Da Capo Press
A Member of the Perseus Books Group
www.dacapopress.com

Note: The information in this book is true and complete to the best of our knowledge. This book is intended only as an informative guide for those wishing to know more about pregnancy. In no way is this book intended to replace, countermand or conflict with the advice given to you by your own physician. The ultimate decision concerning your care should be made between you and your doctor. We strongly recommend that you follow his or her advice. The information in this book is general and is offered with no guarantees on the part of the authors or Da Capo Press. The authors and publisher disclaim all liability in connection with the use of this book. The names and identifying details of people associated with events described in this book have been changed. Any similarity to actual persons is coincidental.

Da Capo Press books are available at special discounts for bulk purchases in the U.S. by corporations, institutions, and other organizations. For more information, please contact the Special Markets Department at the Perseus Books Group, 11 Cambridge Center, Cambridge, MA 02142, or call (800) 255-1514 or (617) 252-5298, or e-mail special.markets@perseusbooks.com.

  3 4 5 6 7 8 9—08 07 06 05 04

CAUTION

Do not begin any exercise program during or immediately after your pregnancy without checking first with your doctor. He or she may have special precautions for you, or you may be advised not to exercise.

Remember—it's for the good of you and your baby!

Find It Fast!

Exercise during Pregnancy

Do you like to exercise? Is it part of your daily routine? Now that you're pregnant, are you wondering if you'll have to give it up?

- If your pregnancy is low risk and you have no medical or physical problems that keep you from exercising, you may be able to continue with a modified exercise routine.
- Discuss it with your doctor at your first prenatal visit.
- Most medical experts agree that exercise during pregnancy is safe and beneficial for most pregnant women, if it is done properly.
- Exercise can help you feel more energetic and help you deal more effectively with the demands of pregnancy, career and family.
- Exercise is an important part of life for many women.
- The more we learn about health, the more the advantages of regular exercise become evident.
- Regular exercise may decrease your risk of developing several medical problems during your lifetime, including cardiovascular disease, osteoporosis (soft-

ening of bones), depression, premenstrual syndrome (PMS) and obesity.

- If you've been reaping the benefits of exercise before pregnancy, you probably want to continue during pregnancy. In addition, you'll reap great pregnancy benefits!
- The goal of exercising during pregnancy is overall good health. It will make you feel better physically, and it can also give you an emotional boost.
- If you get the go-ahead from your doctor, make daily exercise a part of your pregnancy.

The Benefits of Exercise

People used to think that exercise could cause a woman to go into labor too early. We have found in a normal pregnancy that this does not happen. The medical community has realized that exercising during pregnancy can be very beneficial for a pregnant woman and her growing baby.

- Most doctors encourage their pregnant patients to exercise if the pregnancy is low risk, there are no complications and the woman is able to exercise.
- If you exercise throughout your pregnancy, you may see many benefits!
- Regular, moderate exercise during pregnancy can help you in many ways.

- Some of the many benefits of exercising during pregnancy include:
  - ~ relieving backache
  - ~ preventing constipation and varicose veins
  - ~ helping you feel better about yourself
  - ~ lowering your risk of pre-eclampsia and gestational diabetes
  - ~ managing your weight
  - ~ sleeping better
  - ~ helping to prevent some forms of stomach upset
  - ~ lessening fatigue, stress, dizziness and back pain
  - ~ controlling mood swings
  - ~ strengthening muscles needed for delivery
  - ~ carrying baby at least 37 weeks, which results in a healthier baby
  - ~ less need for inducing labor
  - ~ less pain medication needed during labor
  - ~ fewer episiotomies, C-sections and forceps deliveries
  - ~ shorter labor
  - ~ you're in better shape after delivery
- Studies show women who exercise during the first and second trimesters are less likely to have a preterm birth than women who don't exercise at all during pregnancy.

- Exercise may help you have an easier time with your labor and delivery, and a shorter recovery time after birth.
- Pregnant women who exercise may get their prepregnancy shapes back sooner. They also have more energy and deal with stress better after baby's birth.
- Studies show women who did mild weight-bearing exercise during pregnancy had bigger babies than women who didn't exercise.
- If you exercise regularly during pregnancy, it's easier to get back into an exercise program after delivery.
- In the past, exercise was not always approved for a pregnant woman. Doctors were concerned about blood flow to the fetus when the mom-to-be exercised. We now know this happens somewhat but doesn't hurt the baby.
- When you exercise, it forces water in the tissues back into the blood and helps pump blood back to the heart. If your ankles or legs swell, exercise can help with the problem.

If You Exercise Regularly

Many women love to exercise, and they juggle hectic schedules to fit it into their daily routine. Do you feel this way, too? You may feel that exercise (whether or not you are pregnant) is necessary to help you feel good, control your weight and look your best. You don't want to give up exercising just because you're pregnant.

If your pregnancy is uncomplicated, you should be able to exercise as long as you're comfortable. Don't be afraid that exercising might hurt your growing baby; most moderate exercise is safe. However, you may find you need to set new exercise goals and to take things a little easier during pregnancy.

- Most experts recommend reducing exercise to 70 to 80% of your prepregnancy level.
- The goal of exercising at this time is overall good health, but don't overdo it.
- Now is *not* the time to try to set new records or to train for an upcoming marathon!
- If you decide to change your current exercise program, be sure to talk with your physician *before* you do.
- You may also have to change or to modify your exercise program during pregnancy because of changes in your body.
- Your center of gravity shifts, so you may need to adjust your exercise for that.
- As your tummy gets bigger, you may not be able to do some activities very comfortably, and you may have to eliminate others.

- During pregnancy, your heart rate is higher; you don't have to exercise as vigorously to reach your target-heart-rate range. See the discussion of target heart rates on page 13.
- Be careful not to put too much stress on your cardiovascular system.
- If your heart rate gets too high, slow down but don't stop completely. Continue exercising at a moderate rate.
- If your heart rate is too low and you don't feel winded, pick up the pace a bit, but don't overdo it.
- Check your pulse rate frequently to make sure you aren't working too hard.
- It's important not to get too hot during exercise, for the health of your baby.
- Avoid raising your body temperature above 102F. Aerobic exercise can raise your body temperature higher than this, so be careful. Be aware that a high body temperature can go even higher if you're dehydrated.
- Sports drinks may help replenish fluids lost during exercise. They contain electrolytes to help replace those you lose when you sweat. Choose low-sodium drinks when you can.
- Keeping cool is important. Exercise can improve your body's ability to cool itself, but hot conditions and heavy clothes can work against you.

- Choose clothing that breathes, such as cotton. Some of the new, high-tech fabrics wick water away to help keep you cool.
- During hot periods, exercise in the morning or work out inside, at home or at the gym.
- If it's cold, wear several layers of light clothing that you can remove as you get warmer.

If You've Never Exercised Before

Some women don't like to exercise or don't exercise on a regular basis. When many of these women learn they're pregnant, they begin to think about the benefits of exercise. They want to know whether it is safe to begin an exercise program during pregnancy. **If you've never exercised before, you *must* discuss it with your doctor before you begin.**

If your doctor says it's OK to exercise, start with *moderate* exercise.

If you've never exercised before, you may find it difficult to begin because of less flexibility and tighter muscles. However, it is possible to start exercising now, but you have to begin gradually.

- Walking (inside or outside) is a great choice.
- Riding a stationary bike or walking on a treadmill can be enjoyable.

- Swimming and other water exercises may be the most enjoyable, especially as you get bigger. The water provides your body with a lot of support, and you'll also feel a lot lighter in the water.
- See also the discussion of good exercise activities that begins on page 21.

Exercise in the 1st Trimester

- Exercising during the 1st trimester may be difficult for you if you suffer from morning sickness.
- If you don't feel well, don't force yourself to exercise. It's more important to rest and to hold on to the strength you do have at this time.
- If you do feel like exercising, be sure to drink lots of water. It's one of the most important things you can do whenever you exercise.
- Don't increase your workout; take it easy.
- Keep your body temperature below 100F, and keep your heart rate below 140 beats per minute (bpm). See the discussion of target heart rate on page 13.

Exercise in the 2nd Trimester

- You may feel eager to exercise now, especially if you had morning sickness during the 1st trimester. Many women say this is the best time during pregnancy for exercise and other activities!

- As your baby grows and your tummy gets larger, your sense of balance may be affected, and you may feel clumsy. It's normal.
- This isn't the time for contact sports, such as basketball, or sports where you might fall, injure yourself or be struck in the tummy.
- Now is not the time to train for any sport or to increase your activity level. In fact, this may be a good time to decrease the amount or intensity of exercise you are doing.
- Listen to your body. It will tell you when it's time to slow down.

Exercise in the 3rd Trimester

- As you enter this phase of your pregnancy, you may not feel like exercising.
- Your increased weight and the large size of your tummy may make many exercises difficult or uncomfortable for you.
- Exercising in the water may the best form of exercise to do during the 3rd trimester.
- In the water, you have little fear of falling because the water supports you so well.

- You can also get a good workout because the water offers resistance.
- You'll feel light as a feather in the water—you feel as if you weigh only 10% of your weight in water. There's also less stress on joints.

Your Exercise Experience during Pregnancy

- You may notice changes in how your body responds to exercise during pregnancy.
- Your growing tummy can put a strain on your respiratory system, so you may feel out of breath sooner than usual.
- When you exercise, don't work to the point that you can't talk or have trouble breathing. At that point, you're working too hard. Cut back on your workout.
- Don't get overheated during your workout. Work out in a well-ventilated room, and drink lots of water while you exercise.
- Not every place is a good place to exercise. If you're in an area over 8000 feet, don't exercise. It takes about 4 days to acclimate yourself if you're at an altitude over 6500 feet, so take it easy.
- To prevent low blood-sugar levels, eat a piece of fruit or toast, or drink a glass of juice 30 to 60 minutes before exercising.

- Always be sure exercise equipment is in proper working order to avoid injuries.
- You may be getting a lot of exercise just by following your daily routine. Climbing stairs, walking the dog and working in the yard provide exercise. Other exercises you may do every day include gardening, raking the lawn, washing the car, hanging out the laundry, and dusting and vacuuming.
- Don't think you have time for exercise? Try the following.
  - ~ Take the stairs; skip the elevator.
  - ~ Walk to see a friend instead of phoning.
  - ~ Don't drive if you can walk where you want to go.
  - ~ Wash the car yourself.
  - ~ Park at the edge of the parking lot.
  - ~ Lose the remote—get up to change the channel.

General Exercise Guidelines

Before beginning any exercise program, consult your doctor about any medical problems or pregnancy problems. Get his or her OK *before* you begin.

- Allow enough time to warm up; start your exercise routine with a 5-minute warm-up.

- Begin exercising gradually. Start with 10-minute workout sessions, with 5-minute rest periods in between. Work up to longer workout sessions.
- Don't exercise strenuously for more than 15 to 20 minutes.
- Always end with a 5-minute cool-down period. Cool down and stretch your muscles to prevent injury, soreness and stiffness.
- Try to exercise at least 3 times a week for 20 to 30 minutes each time. Work out more often when you can.
- It may be easier to fit several small workouts into your day rather than one long one. Break your exercise time down into manageable segments. Two 15-minute workouts or three 10-minute sessions, 3 to 4 times a week, is good for your body and spirit.
- Take your pulse every 15 minutes. Don't let it go higher than 140 beats per minute (bpm). If your heart rate is higher than 140 beats a minute, rest until your pulse drops below 90 bpm.
- Don't get overheated.
- Wear comfortable clothing when you exercise, including clothing that is warm enough or cool enough for the season and your activity level, a good support bra or a sports bra, and comfortable athletic shoes that offer maximum support.

- Be careful about getting up and lying down.
- Rise slowly from the floor or from a sitting position to avoid getting dizzy.
- After the 4th month of pregnancy (16 weeks), don't lie on your back while exercising. This can decrease blood flow to the uterus and placenta.
- When you finish exercising, lie on your left side for 15 to 20 minutes.
- Don't exercise in hot, humid weather.
- Exercise during the coolest part of the day.
- Stop immediately and consult your physician if you experience any problems. See also the discussion on page 17 in Precautions about Exercising during Pregnancy.
- Modify your exercise routine as needed as your pregnancy progresses.
- Always practice good posture.

Target Heart Rates

- During pregnancy, your heart rate is higher, so you don't have to exercise as hard to reach your target-heart-rate range. Don't stress your cardiovascular system.
- The baby's heart rate does increase somewhat during and immediately after exercise, but it stays within the normal fetal range of 120 to 160 beats a

minute. This shouldn't cause any problems for you or the baby.

- During pregnancy, don't work out as hard as you normally do. Experts suggest 70 to 80% of your prepregnancy effort is fine. This level can still have an effect on your heart rate.

- If your heart rate gets too high, slow down but don't stop exercising completely. Continue exercising, but slow it down.

- If you don't feel too winded, pick up the pace a bit, but again don't overdo it. Recheck your pulse rate in a few minutes to make sure you aren't working too hard.

- During pregnancy, check your heart rate fairly often when you exercise. You may be surprised to see how fast your pulse can increase during a pregnancy workout.

- Keep your heart rate under 140 bpm during a workout.

- Check your heart rate with the following steps. Use a watch with a second hand, or have a clock with a second hand in view.

  ~ Place the index and middle fingers of one hand on the side of your neck where you can feel your pulse.

  ~ After finding your pulse, watch the second hand until it reaches the 12.

~ Begin counting the pulse beats until the second hand reaches the 2 (10 seconds).

~ Multiply that number by 6 to find your heart rate.

Target Heart Rates		
Age (years)	Target heart rate (beats/minute)	Max. heart rate (beats/minute)
20	150	200
25	117–146	195
30	114–146	190
35	111–138	185
40	108–135	180
45	105–131	175
50	102–131	170

(SOURCE: *U.S. Department of Health and Human Services*)

Your Nutritional Needs When You Exercise

Your nutritional needs increase during pregnancy. You will also burn extra calories during exercise so you need to eat enough calories to get a balanced diet. You may need to eat more than a pregnant woman who isn't exercising at your level. Discuss how much more you should eat with your doctor.

• Make sure that any additional calories you eat are nutritious and supply your body with protein, calcium and carbohydrates, not sugar and fat.

- A normal-weight woman often needs to eat between 300 and 800 extra calories a day during pregnancy. Exercising may increase those needs.
- You may need to do *less* exercise, if you burn too many calories when you exercise.
- When you exercise, drink a cup of water before you begin your routine.
- Drink ½ cup to 1 cup of water every 20 minutes during exercise to help prevent dehydration.
- Fluid intake can also help regulate body temperature.
- You may feel better during your pregnancy if you drink more water than you normally do.
- Thirst is *not* a good indication of how much water you need. By the time you get thirsty, you've already lost 1% of your body's water. Don't let yourself become thirsty!

Muscle Strength

Some women exercise for muscle strength; you'll need strong muscles to do the work of labor and delivery. There are various ways to strengthen your muscles.

- To strengthen a muscle, there has to be resistance against it.
- There are three different kinds of muscle exercises—isotonic, isometric and isokinetic.

- *Isotonic exercise* involves shortening the muscle as tension is developed, such as when you lift a weight.
- *Isometric exercise* causes the muscle to develop tension but doesn't change its length, such as when you push against a stationary wall.
- *Isokinetic exercise* occurs when the muscle moves at a constant speed, such as when you swim.
- Strengthening skeletal muscles requires lifting heavy weights, but you should be careful about lifting heavy weights during pregnancy.
- Weight-bearing exercise may be the most effective way to work your muscles during pregnancy. Aerobic exercise is a good weight-bearing exercise to do.
- Many women do both muscle-building *and* aerobic exercises.
- Stretching and warming up muscles before and after exercise help improve flexibility and avoid injury.

Precautions about Exercising during Pregnancy

A few general guidelines about exercising during pregnancy apply to most pregnant women. Your doctor may want to discuss additional precautions that apply specifically to you. You may want to pick an activity to participate in during pregnancy that is not too strenuous.

Whatever you choose, don't get carried away or overwork yourself.

- Stop exercising and consult your doctor if you experience bleeding or loss of fluid from the vagina while exercising.
- Shortness of breath, dizziness, severe abdominal pain or any other pain or discomfort may also be signs of problems.
- Consult your doctor, and exercise only under his or her supervision, if you experience (or know you have) an irregular heartbeat, high blood pressure, diabetes, thyroid disease, anemia or any other chronic medical problem.
- If you experience any of the following symptoms during pregnancy, you may not be able to exercise:
  - ~ high blood pressure early in pregnancy
  - ~ multiple fetuses
  - ~ diagnosed heart disease
  - ~ pre-eclampsia
  - ~ vaginal bleeding
  - ~ a history of an incompetent cervix, preterm labor or repeated miscarriages
- Be aware of problems that might develop while you exercise.
- If you notice any unusual occurrences, report them to your doctor immediately. Be careful about the following:

- ~ pain
- ~ bleeding
- ~ dizziness
- ~ extreme shortness of breath
- ~ palpitations
- ~ loss of fluid from the vagina
- ~ faintness
- ~ abnormally rapid heart rate
- ~ back pain
- ~ pubic pain
- ~ difficulty walking
- ~ breathlessness that doesn't go away
- ~ chest pain
- ~ loss of fetal movement
- Talk to your doctor about exercise if you have a history of three or more miscarriages, an incompetent cervix, intrauterine-growth restriction, premature labor or any abnormal bleeding during pregnancy.

Are There Risks to Exercising during Pregnancy?

- Your growing tummy can put a strain on your respiratory system, causing you to feel out of breath sooner than normal. When you exercise, don't work to the point that you aren't able to talk easily and have trouble breathing. If you can't speak a full sentence comfortably, it means you're working too hard; cut back on your workout.

- When you're pregnant, you may feel warmer than usual. You'll feel warmer, too, when you exercise, so avoid getting too hot during workouts.
- The increased hormone levels and weight gain of pregnancy can make your joints more susceptible to injury. Avoid full situps, double-leg raises and straight-leg toe touches.
- The fetal heart rate increases somewhat during and immediately after exercise, but it stays within the normal fetal range of 120 to 160 beats a minute. A moderate exercise program should not cause any problems for you or your baby.
- If you perspire profusely (and it is not normal for you), you're overdoing it. You may be in danger of overheating. Slow down.
- After 16 weeks of pregnancy, do not do any exercise that requires you to lie flat on your back. When you do this, you reduce the blood supply to the baby.
- Avoid the following sports activities during pregnancy:
  ~ scuba diving
  ~ water skiing
  ~ surfing
  ~ horseback riding
  ~ downhill skiing

~ cross-country skiing
~ riding on a snowmobile or a jet ski
~ any contact sport

Good Exercises to Do during Pregnancy

If you're used to participating in a competitive sport, you may be able to continue during pregnancy, but expect to change the level at which you play. The goal is to maintain your fitness and have fun, not to win the game!

Some good exercise and sports activities are listed below. Most are considered OK for women of any age in a normal, low-risk pregnancy:

- walking
- swimming
- low-impact aerobics designed specifically for pregnancy
- water aerobics
- stationary bicycling
- regular cycling (if you're experienced)
- jogging (if you jogged regularly before pregnancy)
- tennis (played moderately)
- yoga (don't lie flat on your back after the 16th week of pregnancy)
- walking on a treadmill
- using a stair stepper or stair climber

- riding a recumbent bike
- using a Nordic Track ski machine

Walking

Walking is one of the best exercises you can do during pregnancy. Even when the weather is bad, you can walk in many places, such as an enclosed shopping mall, to get a good workout. You can begin walking at almost any time during pregnancy, if you don't overdo it. As pregnancy progresses, you may need to decrease your speed and distance. Below are some other things to keep in mind.

- Two miles of walking at a good pace is adequate.
- Break your walks up so you take them throughout the day, not just in the morning or evening. You'll feel better after each short jaunt.
- During your 1st trimester, when you may feel very tired, try to take a short walk in the morning. In the evening, when you have more time, take a longer stroll. Include your partner for some "couple time."
- In the second trimester, when energy levels may be more normal, alternate your walking routine. Take some leisurely strolls, but also add shorter, more intense walks.
- A 20-minute walk during lunch may boost your energy and help you get through the afternoon.

- When you get closer to delivery, several short walks each day may be more beneficial than a longer walk.
- Whenever you walk, pick a safe route. Later in pregnancy, try to avoid hilly terrain.
- In your 3rd trimester, hiking shoes may offer better ankle support than running shoes.
- A walking plan is a good idea, especially if you've never exercised much before. The plan below is a good one to follow.
    - ~ Walk at least 3 times a week—6 times a week is best.
    - ~ Begin with 10 minutes, and add 5 minutes to each session every week. Build up to a walk of between 30 and 60 minutes.
    - ~ Don't just stroll along. Walk briskly enough so you feel comfortably challenged.
    - ~ Posture is important. Keep your head up, your shoulders back and hold your tummy in (as much as possible).
    - ~ Elbows should be bent; roll your foot from heel to toe.
    - ~ Always stretch after walking.
- By midpregnancy, your feet may be changing and growing. You may need to buy different walking shoes to accommodate the changes.

- Listen to your body, and slow your pace when you need to.

Swimming and Water Exercises

Some women say that while they are pregnant, the only time they really feel comfortable is in the water. If you swim, swim throughout pregnancy. If you have been involved in water exercises (exercising in the shallow end of a swimming pool), you can probably continue this throughout your pregnancy as well. These are exercises you can begin at any time during pregnancy, if you don't overdo it.

- Being in the water has a calming effect on some women, and it can help reduce swelling related to pregnancy.
- Because the water supports you, you will feel much lighter, and you won't have to worry about keeping your balance.
- The water also supports the baby's weight; this can help relieve some of your lower back stress.
- Because you can stand in a more-relaxed posture, you may enjoy a greater range of motion while in the water.
- Being in the water reduces the effect of gravity, which in turn reduces pressure on your joints—a great temporary relief for some women.

- Exercising in the water makes it easier for your heart to pump blood. That's a real benefit, especially if you have high blood pressure.
- You can get a good workout in the water. Water exerts 12 times the resistance of air on limbs, so you expend more energy moving through water than you would walking down the street.
- Don't be concerned about water getting to the baby. Baby is well protected inside your body while you're in the water. There are actually three barriers that provide protection—the amniotic membrane that surrounds the baby, the cervix and the vagina.
- However, if your bag of waters has broken, do not exercise in the water.
- Be sure pool water is warm enough to be comfortable but not too hot (nor too cold).
- The ideal temperature of the water should be between 80 and 84F.
- Avoid hot tubs and spas because water is too hot for the fetus.
- Drink plenty of fluids before you begin exercising and during exercise. Dehydration can occur even in a pool.
- Eat easily digested foods ½ to 1 hour before you work out; choose fruit or a whole-grain product.

- To help you keep your footing when you exercise in the pool, wear aquatic shoes, tennis shoes or jogging shoes. Be sure the shoe has a good tread so you don't slip.

Cycling

For some women, cycling is a very enjoyable sport. It allows them to get outside, to breathe fresh air and to get a change of scenery while they exercise. If you're comfortable riding and have safe places to ride, you can enjoy this exercise with your partner or family. However, now is not the time to learn to ride a bike.

- Your balance will change as your body changes. This can make getting on and off a bicycle difficult.
- A fall from a bicycle could injure you or your baby.
- A stationary bicycle is good for bad weather and for later in pregnancy. Many doctors suggest you ride a stationary bike in the last 3 to 4 months of pregnancy to avoid the danger of a fall.
- The weight of your tummy can cause lower-back pain, which may make it very uncomfortable to ride a bike. A recumbent bike may be a better choice, especially for the added back support.

Aerobic Exercise

For cardiovascular fitness, aerobic exercise is the best. If you exercised aerobically before pregnancy, you can probably continue aerobic exercise at a somewhat slower pace. However, it is unwise to start a strenuous aerobic exercise program or to increase training during pregnancy. Aerobics classes designed for pregnant women are a good choice. They concentrate on your unique needs, such as strengthening tummy muscles and improving posture.

- When doing aerobic exercise, don't work as hard as you normally do to avoid potential problems.
- You must exercise at least 3 times a week at a sustained heart rate of 110 to 120 beats a minute, maintained for at least 15 continuous minutes. (The rate of 110 to 120 beats a minute is an approximate target for people of different ages.)
- If you have any problems, such as bleeding or premature labor, you may have to avoid aerobic exercise. Discuss with your doctor another form of exercise.
- If you can't find a pregnancy aerobics class, make some changes in your normal workout. Switch to a low-impact class.
- If you like step aerobics, lower your step; don't step higher than 4 inches.
- Avoid jumps and abrupt moves. Don't twist and turn too much.
- When choosing a class, be sure the instructor has proper training and the class meets the exercise guidelines developed by the American College of

Obstetricians and Gynecologists (ACOG). To obtain a copy of the guidelines, write to:

ACOG Exercise Program
4021 Rosewood Ave.
Los Angeles, CA 90004
(1-213-383-2862)

Other Exercise and Sports Activities

Pilates

- Pilates is a low-impact fitness method that strengthens and lengthens various muscles, which can result in a stronger pelvic floor, increased stamina and other benefits during pregnancy.
- The program can help prepare you for birth by strengthening muscles used during labor and by increasing muscle stamina.
- Be sure your Pilates instructor has experience training pregnant women.
- You may have to modify some of the exercises you perform. Remember to avoid exercises that require you to lie on your back after 16 weeks of pregnancy.

Golf

- If you golf, ask your doctor about playing while you're pregnant.

- If you've never played golf before, you may want to wait until after baby's birth to begin.
- Body changes may change your game. Your balance may be affected, and you may have less endurance.
- If your ligaments loosen, which often happens during pregnancy, you may be more susceptible to injury when playing golf.
- Be sure to warm up to loosen shoulder and arm muscles before you play.
- Drink lots of water or a sports drink while you're on the golf course. Have snacks on hand.
- Don't play if it is hot—either play when it's cool or don't play at all.
- Watch your balance; if you become too unstable, don't play.
- If the course is long, take a cart.
- Consider playing only nine holes after the 5th month of pregnancy.

Tennis
- If you're in good physical shape as you enter pregnancy, discuss with your doctor, at one of your first prenatal visits, if you can play tennis.
- If you get the OK to play tennis, take extra good care of yourself when you play.
- Drink lots of fluids while you're on the court.

- Stop often to drink water or a sports drink.
- Avoid playing in the hot sun—play inside or play early or late, when it's not so hot.
- Wear good-fitting shoes. The shoes you wore before pregnancy may not fit your foot well as pregnancy progresses. You may have to buy larger or wider shoes if your feet change during pregnancy.
- Wear a good sports bra that supports your growing breasts.
- Loose-fitting cotton clothes may be the most comfortable. Some of the new high-tech fabrics that wick away perspiration are good choices.
- Layer clothes if the weather is cool.
- You will probably have to adapt your game as you get larger.
- You may want to play only doubles, so you don't have to run as much.
- Skip the overhead shots and the hard serves. Turning or twisting sharply to reach a ball is not a good idea. Let those go by.
- You may even want to let the ball take a couple of bounces so you don't have to rush around the court.
- Be careful of ankle sprains and strains as ligaments loosen.

Strength Training

- Also called *weight lifting,* strength training can help you prepare for labor and delivery, and it may pay off with the added strength you'll need to lift and carry baby after birth.
- If you want to do strength training during pregnancy, check with your doctor at one of your first prenatal visits. He or she may have precautions for you.
- If you get the go-ahead, lift only a comfortable amount of weight.
- Never overdo it—decrease the weight and do more repetitions if you find yourself getting winded.

Yoga

- Yoga can be especially beneficial for a pregnant woman because it can help keep you fit and flexible.
- In addition, the focus on meditation during yoga can help relieve stress you may experience during your pregnancy.
- A prenatal yoga class is a good choice. The class will teach you moves to accommodate your growing tummy.
- The strength you gain from doing yoga exercises may help make your labor and delivery easier.

- Some cautions—don't hold a posture so long that you overstretch.
- In the 2nd trimester, avoid backbends, inverted postures and jumping into poses.
- Don't do any exercises or movements after the 16th week that require you to lie flat on your back.

Some yoga-type exercises can be fun to do together at home, as a couple. They help improve your balance and flexibility. They can also help tone your muscles.

- In the first exercise, stand about a foot apart, facing each other. Grasp each other's wrists. Breathing deeply, each of you should gently lean back as far as it is comfortable to do so. Hold this position for at least 10 seconds, then slowly come back to an upright position. Repeat several times.
- In the next exercise, stand side by side, with your feet about 10 to 12 inches away from your partner, your arms around each other's waists and your hips touching. Lift your outside foot, and place the bottom of it against the inside of your inner thigh while your partner helps stabilize you. Breathe deeply while your partner supports you in this position. Repeat several times, then turn around and do the exercise with the other leg.
- In the third exercise, sit on the floor facing one another. Stretch legs apart, and touch the soles of your

feet to the soles of your partner's feet. Holding each other's arms, breathe deeply for up to 60 seconds while you maintain the stretch.

Jogging or Running

- If you are used to jogging and have been involved in regular jogging before pregnancy, you may be able to continue to jog in moderation during pregnancy. But check with your doctor first.
- Listen to your body when it tells you to slow down—don't get overheated, stop if you feel tired and drink lots of water.
- Jogging may be permitted during pregnancy, but if your pregnancy is high risk, this exercise may not be a good idea.
- Pregnancy is not the time to increase mileage or to train for a race.
- Wear comfortable clothing and supportive athletic shoes with good cushioning.
- Allow plenty of time to cool down.
- During the course of your pregnancy, you'll probably need to slow down and to decrease the number of miles you run. You may even change to a combination of running and walking. Toward the end of pregnancy, you may want to switch to walking.

- If you notice pain, contractions, bleeding or other symptoms during or after jogging, call your doctor immediately.

Massage Techniques to Relieve Pregnancy Discomforts

- Massaging away tiredness and fatigue can feel great during pregnancy. Massage can also help relieve stress and ease tension, which could help lower your blood pressure. Many of these benefits come from improved blood circulation.
- Massage can benefit you by helping to relieve common pregnancy discomforts, such as fatigue, back pain, sciatica, swelling, constipation, headaches, muscle cramps and varicose veins.
- One study showed that pregnant women who received two 20-minute massages a week for 5 weeks had improved moods, slept better and experienced less back pain. And the babies born to these women had fewer complications.
- You may enjoy having your feet or hands massaged to help relieve swelling and to help your joints move more easily. Ask your partner to give you a hand or foot massage.
- A foot massage can do more than just make your feet feel good. When your feet are massaged, you

may find relief from headaches, higher energy levels and better digestion!

- Acupressure, an ancient form of massage, can also help relieve common discomforts.
- You don't have to get a professional massage to reap the benefits. You can perform some massage techniques yourself. For example, you can massage your legs or your feet to help with swelling.
- Sometimes your aches are too far away for you to reach comfortably. At other times, your pains are completely out of reach.
- Ask your partner to participate in a massage. It can also help you both by strengthening your couple bond.
- One way to get started is to find some books or rent some videos that show various massage techniques. Some are available that focus mainly on pregnant women.
- Neither you nor your partner need to be an expert; take your time and concentrate on doing the best you can.
- As you both practice the kneading and stroking techniques, you'll get better at doing them.
- Gentle pressure should always be used.
- Use massage oil (you can buy this at a drugstore or discount store) or a heavy moisturizer. Massage oil

might be better to use because it stands up better to friction.

- When your partner gives you a massage, find a warm, quiet area, away from drafts.
- Don't have a massage immediately after a meal; wait at least an hour.
- Pillows and a blanket can help make you more comfortable and support your growing tummy.
- Keep in mind that you shouldn't lie flat on your back after 16 weeks of pregnancy. You can partially recline or lie on your side for a massage.
- Don't let anyone put pressure directly on your tummy.
- After your partner gives you a massage, offer to give him one. It's only fair. And when you give a massage, it can help reduce any swelling in your hands!
- If you must be on bed rest, your inactivity could result in muscle pain and weakening. Massage can help relieve these problems.

Backache Relief

- Many women experience back pain during pregnancy. It's one of the most common discomforts women report they have.
- Back pain is often caused by relaxing ligaments that put added strain on your back muscles.

- A pregnant woman's overstretched tummy muscles also put stress on the back as they attempt to support her upper and middle body.
- Having a back massage can work wonders for you.

Help Reduce Swelling

- In addition to relieving discomfort, massage can help with swelling.
- If your legs are swollen, ask your partner to give you a massage to help relieve the swelling. If your hands are swollen, a hand massage can feel great and help reduce swelling.
- Lie on your side on the sofa or bed. Place a pillow or two under your head. Have your partner sit by your feet, and place your legs in his lap. Ask him to begin on the leg that is on top. In one long, gliding movement done with his entire hand flat on your body, have him move his hand along your thigh, from your knee to your hip, on the front of your leg. Ask him to do this several times, then have him do the same movement on the back of your thigh. Be sure the pressure exerted is toward your heart, which helps move fluid out of your extremities.
- Next, while gently pressing and kneading in a circular motion just above your ankle, have him begin making small circles up your leg toward your heart.

- Last, ask him to put his hand under your heel, and lift your top leg a few inches. Have him move his hand up your leg from the Achilles tendon (the tendon that extends from the back of your calf to your heel) to the thigh. Ask him to alternate hands so he massages both sides of your leg.
- When he has finished massaging one leg, roll over onto your other side so he can massage your other leg.

Sciatica Is a Real Pain

- Sciatica can be extremely painful, and massage can help alleviate it.
- Lie on your side on the sofa or bed, with your affected leg on top. Ask your partner to kneel next to you on the floor. Have him apply gentle pressure to the length of your leg in one long, gliding movement done with his entire hand flat on your body. Have him do this to the front of your leg, then the back of the same leg. Have him start with the thigh, then move to your lower leg and end with your foot. Buttocks should be included in the massage.
- Next, your entire leg should be lightly kneaded with one of his hands while his other hand is placed on your hip to stabilize the leg. Repeat several times.

- Last, your partner's thumbs should be placed on the back of your leg, at the top. Both thumbs should be moved together down your leg. Next, in one long, gliding movement done with his entire hand flat on your body, your partner should move his hand along the entire length of the back of your leg. Finally, he should tap the back of your thigh near your buttocks with the back of his hand for 15 seconds.

Prenatal Exercises to Do at Home or at Work

You may find it difficult to exercise outside your home or at a health club. If so, you can do the exercises in this section at home or at work. You don't need any special equipment, so you can do them when you have some spare time. Try all of them, and incorporate those you like into your regular schedule.

Strengthening with Cans

- Next time you're putting away groceries, work on arm muscles by doing a little weight lifting with each can (water bottles and milk cartons also work well).
- As you put a can away, flex your arm a couple of times to work arm muscles. Alternate arms to give yourself a good workout.

Work Out while Waiting

- While standing in line at the grocery store, post office or anywhere else, use the time to do some "creative" exercises.
- These exercises help you develop and strengthen some of the muscles you'll use during labor and delivery.
- Rise up and down on your toes to work your calves.
- Spread your feet apart slightly, and do subtle side lunges to give quadriceps a workout.
- Clench and relax buttocks muscles.
- Do some Kegel exercises (see page 42) to strengthen vaginal muscles.
- Tighten and hold in tummy muscles.

Stand and Stretch

- If you're forced to stand in one place for a long time, step forward slightly with one foot. Place all your weight on that foot for a few minutes.
- If you're still waiting, do the same with the other foot. Alternate the leg you begin with each time.
- This exercise helps stretch leg muscles. Do it when you've been sitting a long time, such as at your desk or in a car or on a plane.

Stretching Reaches

- You probably have to reach for things at home or at the office. When you do, make it an exercise in controlled breathing.
- Before you stretch, inhale, rise up on your toes and bring both arms up at the same time.
- When you're finished, drop back on your heels.
- Exhale while slowly returning your arms to your sides.

Rest and Breathe

- Anytime you are sitting quietly—at home, at the office, in your car, on a bus or a train—do this breathing exercise to strengthen abdominal muscles.
- Breathe deeply and contract stomach muscles; hold for 3 seconds, then exhale slowly. Do this whenever you get the chance.

Backache-Relief Bend

- While standing at the kitchen counter or a counter at work, bend your knees and lean forward from your hips. Hold the position for a few minutes.
- This exercise is an excellent way to relieve back stress.

Graceful Rise

- Some women find it difficult to get out of a chair gracefully during pregnancy.
- This exercise helps you maintain your grace and is also beneficial for you.
- Use leg muscles to lower yourself into and raise yourself out of a chair.
- When getting up, slide to the front edge of the seat. Using your arms for support, push up with your legs to get out of the chair.

Kegel Exercises

- Kegel exercises strengthen pelvic muscles and help you relax your muscles for delivery. These exercises can also be helpful in getting vaginal muscles back in shape after delivery of your baby. You can do them anywhere, anytime, without anyone knowing that you're doing them!
- While sitting, contract the lowest muscles of your pelvis as tightly as you can.
- Tighten muscles higher in the pelvis in stages until you reach the muscles at the top.
- Count to 10 slowly as you move up the pelvis.
- Hold briefly, then release slowly in stages, counting to 10 again. Repeat 2 or 3 times a day.

- You can also do Kegels by tightening the pelvic muscles first, then tightening the anal muscle.
- Hold for a few seconds, then release slowly, in reverse order.
- To see if you're doing these exercises correctly, stop the flow of urine the next time you go to the bathroom. When you do this, you're using the pelvic muscles involved in the Kegel exercises.

Controlled Breathing

- Breathing exercises you do during pregnancy may help during labor.
- Using your diaphragm muscles to breathe is beneficial to you. These are the muscles you will use during labor and delivery.
- Breath training decreases the amount of energy you need to breathe, and it improves the function of your respiratory muscles.
- Practice the different breathing exercises below for benefits in the near future (labor and delivery!).
- Breathe in through your nose, and exhale through pursed lips. Making a little whistling sound is OK. Breathe in for 4 seconds, and breathe out for 6 seconds.
- Lie back, propped on some pillows, in a comfortable position. Place your hand on your tummy

while breathing. If you breathe using your diaphragm, your hand will move up when you inhale and down when you exhale. If it doesn't, try using different muscles until you can do it correctly.

- Bend forward to breathe. If you bend slightly forward, you'll find it's easier to breathe. If you feel pressure as your baby gets bigger, try this technique. It may offer some relief.

Modified Crunches

- By now, you know you shouldn't exercise lying flat on your back after the 16th week. That means no crunches.
- To help strengthen stomach muscles and keep your lower back and spine strong, try this exercise.
- Sit on the floor in a crossed-leg position.
- Brace your back against the wall. Use pillows for added comfort.
- Exhaling through your nose, pull your bellybutton in toward your spine.
- Hold for 5 seconds, then exhale through your nose.
- Begin with 5 repetitions and work up to 10.

Your Pregnancy Workout

- Practice the exercises in the previous section, and add the following ones to your routine.
- You may have to set extra time aside to do these exercises.
- If you combine them with some form of aerobic exercise, such as walking, swimming or bicycling, you'll get a good workout.
- If an exercise calls for light weights, and you don't have any, use a can! A 16-ounce can of vegetables or soup can be held in each hand to provide you with some resistance.
- Another way to make a weight is to take a couple of plastic half-gallon juice or milk containers (with handles); clean them out and add water. A pint (16 ounces) weighs about a pound, so 32 ounces would give you a 2-pound weight and 64 ounces (a filled ½-gallon container) would be 4 pounds.

Reach for the Stars

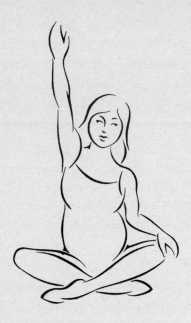

Relieves upper backache and tension in shoulders, neck and back.

Sit on the floor in a comfortable position. Inhale as you raise your right arm over your head. Reach as high as you can, while stretching from the waist. Bend your elbow, and pull your arm back down to your side as you exhale. Repeat for your left side. Do 4 or 5 times on each side.

Tailor's Seat

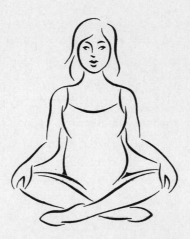

Develops pelvic-floor strength.

Sit on the floor, bring feet close to your body and cross your ankles. Apply gentle pressure to your knees or the inside of your thighs. Hold for a count of 10, relax and repeat. Do this exercise 4 or 5 times.

Seamstress's Press

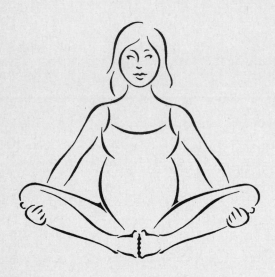

Develops pelvic-floor strength and quadricep strength.

Sit on the floor, and bring the soles of your feet together as close to your body as you comfortably can. Place hands under your knees, and gently press down with your knees while resisting the pressure with your hands. Count to 5, then relax. Increase the number of presses until you can do 10 presses twice a day.

Wall Pusher

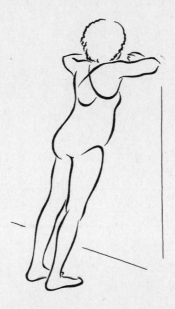

Develops upper-back, chest and arm strength, and relieves lower-leg tension.

Stand a couple of feet away from a wall, with your hands in front of your shoulders. Place hands on the wall, and lean forward. Bend your elbows as your body leans into the wall. Keep heels flat on the floor. Slowly push away from wall, and stand straight. Do 10 to 20 times.

Petal Stretch

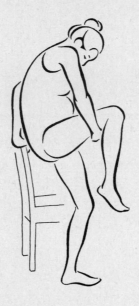

Reduces back tension, and increases blood flow to the feet.

Place your left hand on the back of a chair or against the wall. Lift your right knee up, and put your right hand under your thigh. Round your back, and bring head and pelvis forward. Hold position for count of 4, straighten up, then lower leg. Repeat with left leg. Do 5 to 8 times with each leg.

Leisure Lifts

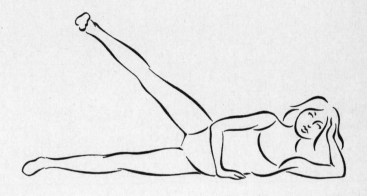

Tones and strengthens hip, buttock and thigh muscles.

Lie on your left side, with your body in alignment. Support your head with your left hand, and place your right hand on the floor in front of you for balance. Inhale and relax. While exhaling, slowly raise your right leg as high as you can without bending your knee or your body. Keep foot flexed. Inhale, and slowly lower your leg. Repeat on right side. Do 10 times on each side.

The Swan

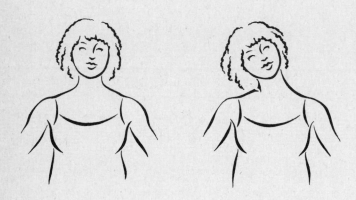

Helps stretch the neck, and relieves neck and shoulder tension.

Sit on a chair or on the floor in a crossed-leg position. Inhale, and slowly tilt your head to the right until you feel a stretch in your neck. Breathe deeply 3 times while holding the stretch. Slowly bring your head to the center, then tilt your head to the left. Hold while you breathe deeply 3 times. Do 4 times on each side.

Wing Stretch

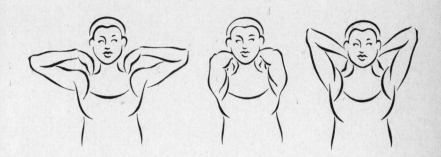

Opens and stretches the back and chest.

Sit on the floor or in a chair, or stand with feet slightly apart. Place your fingers on your shoulders, with elbows pointed out to the side. Bring elbows forward, then lift elbows toward ceiling. Hold for a count of 2. Exhale, lower elbows and return to starting position, with elbows out to the side. Do entire exercise 4 times.

Rani Stretch

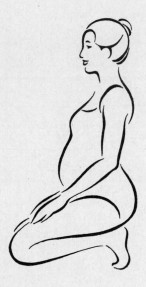

Loosens calf and foot muscles; may help prevent leg cramps.

Kneel on the ground, with feet tucked under you and toes on the ground. Sit tall. Press toes into the ground. Hold. Do 5 or 6 times, or as often as you want.

Gazelle Stretch

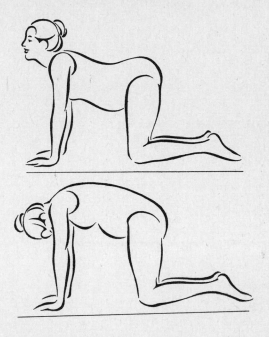

Stretches back and tummy muscles, and increases flexibility.

Kneel on hands and knees, with hands directly below shoulders and knees directly under hips. Inhale as you raise your head and gaze forward. Then exhale as you slowly bring your head down, round your shoulders and tuck in your tummy. Do 4 times.

Opening Flower

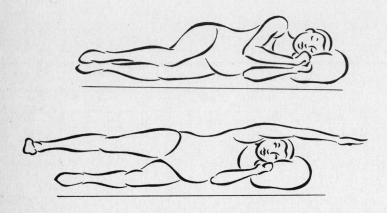

Helps improve posture, and stretches back muscles.

Lie on your left side on the floor or bed. Elevate your head with a pillow. Bend knees, and pull arms close to the body. While inhaling, reach right arm over your head as you fully extend the right leg, leading with the heel. Hold for 3 seconds. Exhale as you return to starting position. Do 4 times on each side.

Soccer Stretch

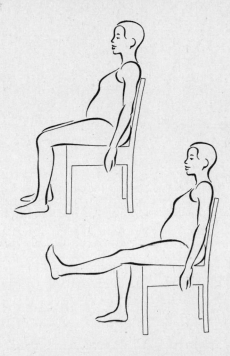

Stretches hamstrings, and strengthens thigh muscles.

Sit tall in a straight-backed side chair, with knees bent, arms relaxed at your side and feet flat on the floor. Lift your left foot off the floor, with the leg extended. Hold for 8 seconds; be sure you are sitting erect. Lower left leg. Do 5 times for each leg.

Fencing Stretch

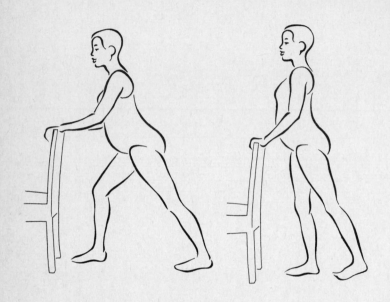

Helps increase circulation and flexibility in the legs.

Place both hands on the back of a chair. Lean forward, keeping left leg on the floor to stretch the calf. Hold for 3 seconds. Bring left leg forward, and stand straight. Keeping right knee slightly bent, extend left leg behind you while keeping foot flexed. Hold for 3 seconds. Do 4 repetitions, then switch legs.

Air Circles

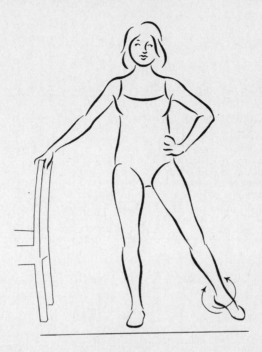

Strengthens hip flexors and pelvic-floor muscles.

While holding on to the back of a chair, raise your right leg so your foot is slightly off the floor. Try to maintain your balance. Make 8 small circles in one direction with your foot, then 8 small circles in the other direction with the same foot. Switch to the left leg and repeat.

Sofa Stretch

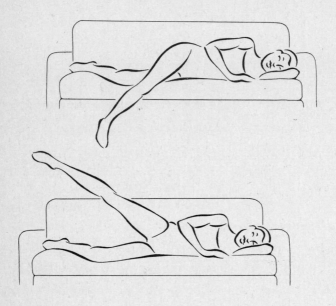

Helps ease sciatica; strengthens hip and upper-buttock muscles.

Lie on your left side on the sofa, with left knee bent. Bend your left arm, and place your head on it. Lower your right foot to the floor while keeping your leg straight. Hold for 10 seconds, then lift the straightened leg to a 45° angle; hold for 5 seconds. Do 5 complete repetitions with each leg.

Tush Taps

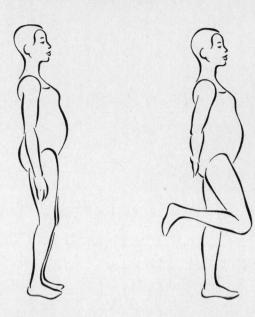

Tones quadriceps.

Stand with feet slightly apart and knees soft. Hold onto a counter or a chair with your left hand for stability, if you need it. Holding in tummy muscles, lift your right leg up behind you, until you can touch your tush (your bottom) with your foot. Return foot to the floor. Turn around, hold onto support with right hand and lift left foot. Repeat 8 times for each leg.

Pat Yourself on the Back

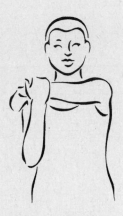

Provides good stretch for upper back.

Stand with feet slightly apart and knees soft. Cross your chest with your right arm. With left hand, gently push your right elbow closer to your chest. Pat yourself on the back for a pregnancy job well done! Hold stretch for 10 seconds; repeat 4 times for each arm.

Arm Swishers

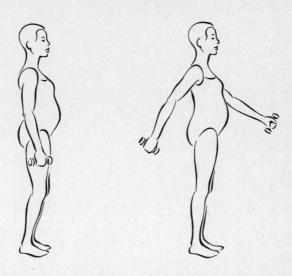

Strengthens upper body.

Stand with feet slightly apart and knees soft. (You can also do this exercise sitting down.) Standing or sitting tall, square shoulders. Hold your tummy in. Using light weights (2 to 3 pounds each to start; if you don't have weights, use a 16-ounce can), slowly raise your left arm straight in front of you. Stop just below shoulder height. Hold for a count of 6. Don't swing your arms; control the movement. Slowly lower your left arm to starting position, then raise right arm. Repeat 10 times for each arm.

The Seagull

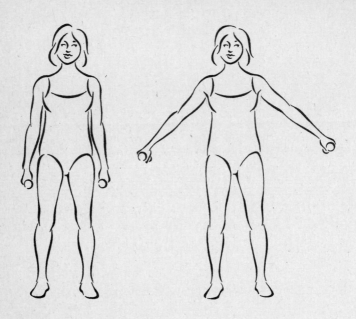

Strengthens upper body.

Stand with feet slightly apart and knees soft, with arms by your side. Hold your tummy in. Using light weights (2 to 3 pounds each to start; if you don't have weights, use a 16-ounce can), raise arms together; stop just below shoulder height. Hold for a count of 4. Don't swing your arms; control the movement. Slowly lower your arms to starting position. Repeat 15 times.

Curling Iron

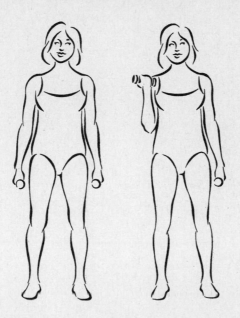

Strengthens arms.

Stand with feet slightly apart and knees soft, with arms by your side. Hold your tummy in. Using light weights (2 to 3 pounds each to start; if you don't have weights, use a 16-ounce can), exhale as you curl your right hand toward your shoulder. Hold for a count of 5. Inhale as you lower your arm to your side, then raise right arm. Repeat 10 times for each arm.

Baby Squats

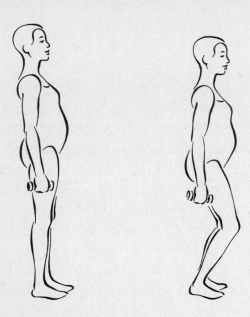

Strengthens quadriceps.

Stand with feet shoulder-width apart and knees soft, with arms by your side. Hold your tummy in. Using light weights (2 to 3 pounds each to start; if you don't have weights, use a 16-ounce can), keep hands by your hips, head up and back straight. Inhale as you squat about 6 inches; hold for 5 seconds. Exhale as you squeeze your buttocks muscles and return to standing position. Repeat 8 times.

After Pregnancy—
Exercise Your Way Back to Fitness

One important question you may have after your baby is born is, "How soon can I start exercising?" After months of watching your body change so dramatically, you may want to get back in shape as soon as possible. You may be eager to begin exercising soon after baby's birth. In addition to helping you get back in shape, exercise can help you feel better and lift your spirits. It can also increase your circulation, help you heal and ease body soreness. It can even give you more energy!

- There are many things you can do to get back in shape—you can do some of them while you're still in the hospital.
- Be sure to ask your doctor or the nurses taking care of you if it's OK to do these activities.
- Start by doing simple exercises immediately after delivery.
- Practice holding your stomach muscles in.
- Do your Kegel exercises (see page 42).
- Even sitting down can be an exercise. If you can sit in a chair, sit tall in the chair. Plant feet firmly on the floor. Align hips and shoulders while sitting straight. Open

your shoulders, and lengthen your neck. Keep head high. Tighten pelvic muscles and tummy muscles.

- When you are up and about in the hospital, you can do other forms of exercise, if you didn't have any complications during the pregnancy or birth that would prevent you from being active.

- When you feel able, get up and walk around the hospital.

- Do mild leg and arm stretches, which may feel very good after delivery. During labor and delivery, you used many muscles, often tensing them during pushing. Stretching after recovery can relieve some tension and loosen your muscles.

- Other exercises you can do include leg stretches, neck and shoulder rolls, shoulder shrugs, and foot and ankle circles.

- If you have done yoga exercises in the past, some of the gentler stretches may be good to do at this time.

- No matter what you do after baby's birth, a word to the wise: Don't expect to leave the hospital in the shape or physical condition you were in before you became pregnant.

Exercise in the Weeks following Birth

Exercise in the weeks following your baby's birth can be important to your feeling of well-being. If you exercised regularly during pregnancy, you may be able to continue with many of the same exercises. Your body is probably still in good condition, so after delivery you may be able to begin exercising sooner and increase your levels a little more quickly. Before you start any postpartum exercise program, check with your doctor. He or she may have particular advice for you.

- Do something you enjoy, and do it on a regular basis.
- Walking and swimming are excellent exercises to help you get back in shape.
- Your aerobic capacity can increase as much as 20% in the 6 weeks following baby's birth. This is good news, especially if you are overly fatigued.
- As your hormones return to normal levels, you'll probably have more energy.
- You may be able to do gentle stretches and take leisurely walks without any problems.
- Your doctor may advise you to let your body be your guide as to how much you can do and how much intensity you can put into your exercising.
- Changes in your cardiovascular system caused by pregnancy can last up to 6 weeks postpartum, which can affect your ability to exercise.
- Keep a positive attitude. Many athletes have found their level of conditioning was better after pregnancy and delivery. There is hope!

- If you can exercise on a regular basis, no matter what the weather is or what kind of interruptions you may experience, you will be more successful in achieving your goal of fitness.
- Exercise helps strengthen underlying tummy muscles, but it won't necessarily give you back your prepregnancy figure.
- How your tummy area looks after pregnancy depends on heredity, your muscle tone, the elasticity of your skin and how much body fat you retain.
- While trying to get back into an exercise routine, take it easy. It may take longer to tone your muscles, and you may also find your body shape has changed due to pregnancy.
- Sometimes it's hard for a new mom to get out of the house to go exercise. If this happens to you, use a videotape to guide you. You can check them out at the library, rent them or buy them.
- Taking baby for a walk—in a front pack or a stroller—is a great way for you and baby to bond and for you to get some exercise.
- If you were on bed rest for longer than 2 weeks before baby's birth, you need to take it easy when beginning an exercise program.
- Studies show that if you spent a prolonged time in bed, you may have suffered significant muscle deterioration.

- If you were in bed longer than 2 or 3 weeks, you may need a physical-therapy assessment. Ask your doctor about it.
- Don't overtire yourself by choosing a program that is too ambitious.

Some Precautions about Exercising after a C-Section

- After a Cesarean delivery, light activity is very important.
- In the hospital, you'll probably have to practice coughing or deep breathing to keep your lungs clear.
- Wiggle toes to aid circulation.
- Walking may be uncomfortable, but it helps minimize the chances of developing a blood clot.
- Check with your doctor before starting an exercise routine or exercise program of any kind. It's important to know that your body has healed and you are ready to exercise.
- It may take longer to get your tummy area back in shape if you had a C-section. You may have to wait until after your 6-week checkup before you can do crunches or other stomach exercises.
- Within 4 weeks, you should be able to start a light-exercise program.
- It may take longer before you can engage in activities that require all-out effort, such as running or

lifting heavy weights. Full recovery could take months.

- If you experience any pain, a significant increase in bleeding or other complications, listen to your body. These problems may be telling you that you haven't fully recovered. You may need to ease up on the level or intensity of your exercise.

Exercising at Home

- Whether you had a vaginal delivery or a C-section, after you get the OK from your doctor, do some sort of exercise that you enjoy. Do it on a regular basis.
- Getting back into shape takes time. It's easy to feel discouraged when you begin because you probably want immediate results.
- As the saying goes, "It took 9 months for your body to get into the shape it is now." Realize it will take some time to get it back into the shape you would like to be in.
- Don't be too hard on yourself, and don't expect miracles.
- It will probably take some planning and dedication on your part to fit an exercise routine into a busy, hectic schedule, but you'll be happy you did when you see positive results.

- You'll have more energy if you exercise, which you probably need now that you have a new baby to take care of!
- Try to plan time for exercise; do some type of aerobic activity for at least 20 to 30 minutes at least 3 times a week (5 times a week is best for getting back in shape).
- Walking and swimming are excellent exercises to help you get back in shape.
- If you want to do water exercises, your doctor will probably advise you to wait until bleeding stops completely, which could take from 3 to 6 weeks.
- Some nonweight-bearing activities are excellent for after-baby fitness, such as riding a stationary bicycle or working out on a stair stepper.
- Mild aerobic exercises, such as light step aerobics, may be started soon after delivery.
- You might be able to begin strengthening exercises, using light weights, soon after your baby's birth. Use 1- or 2-pound weights for arm and leg exercises (use ankle weights for your legs).
- At your 6-week postpartum checkup, talk to your doctor about resuming your normal exercise activities, such as playing tennis or golf, or doing yoga or Pilates routines.

Be a Success!

There are some things you can to do to help yourself be successful in your workouts.

- To lose fat, do some type of aerobic activity, such as biking, running, swimming or aerobic-exercise classes. These exercises use large muscle groups, elevate your heart rate and burn calories, which in turn burns fat your body stored during pregnancy.
- If you can work out 20 to 30 minutes 3 to 5 times a week, you'll find your body will respond.
- You may feel self-conscious about exercising with others if you feel out of shape. Find a class for new mothers, or exercise with someone else who has just had a baby. Or work out when traffic is light at the gym, such as late morning or early afternoon.
- If you can't get out to exercise, an exercise videotape you can buy, rent or check out from the library is another option. There are many on the market specifically for new moms.
- Check out exercise programs on TV. You can work out while baby sleeps.

Tips for Starting Your Exercise Program

- Do something you enjoy. Choose some sort of exercise that you will continue on a regular basis.

- Time may be limited, so use it wisely. If you have the chance to do something while baby sleeps, do it.
- Work out when you can. Two or three 10-minute exercise sessions spread out during the day may be easier to handle than a full 20 or 30 minutes at one time.
- Pay attention to your nutritional needs.
- Don't go on a strict diet in an attempt to lose weight quickly.
- You need adequate nutrition to make breast milk, if you breastfeed.
- Even if you don't breastfeed, your body needs energy to take care of your baby and yourself, so don't skimp on your food. Eat nutritiously.
- Your body has undergone some major changes, so don't be too hard on yourself. You may have to accept these changes because there may not be much you can do about them.
- Avoid the scale and weighing yourself. Instead, let your clothes be your guide.
- Tune in to your body, and check out how you feel. Use these measures as another gauge to determine your progress.
- Work out with a friend, especially another new mom. Walk together or agree to do some other type of activity. Take your babies when possible. If you know someone else depends on you for support, it may be easier to stay committed.

- If you find you're getting bored with your routine or you feel very tired, try to make some positive changes. Try another activity.
- Keep working out, even when you feel exhausted— sometimes exercise can help increase your energy level and make you feel less tired.
- Always warm up and cool down, whether you are doing aerobic exercise or toning exercises. Warm up by walking briskly or marching in place for 5 to 10 minutes. When finished with your activities, cool down by stretching for at least 5 minutes.
- Before you begin exercising, you'll probably need to gather together some things to help make your workout easier and more enjoyable.
- Paying attention to these details before you begin will increase the enjoyment and benefits you will receive from your exercise program.
  - ~ Wear the right clothes and shoes. Clothes should be comfortable and allow your body to "breathe."
  - ~ Wear shoes that offer good support.
  - ~ A sports bra may provide added relief to enlarged and/or sore breasts.
  - ~ Drink lots of water. Start before you exercise, and keep hydrated all during your exercise period.
  - ~ Keep doing your Kegels! (See page 42.)

After-Baby Exercises to Tone Your Body

In this final section, you will find a collection of various isometric and isotonic exercises you can do to help you get back in shape. These exercises help you build or regain strength in your muscles. Aerobic exercise should also be done in addition to these activities because it increases your metabolism and helps burn fat.

Choose exercises from this section that focus on the body areas you want to work on. Try to do these activities at least 3 times a week—every other day helps tone muscles. You might want to alternate aerobic activity and toning exercises from one day to the next.

Continue doing the exercises you did during pregnancy, even after your baby is born. They begin on page 39. Add some of the exercises that follow to help you focus on specific areas, especially your tummy. Remember, do not begin these exercises until your doctor gives you permission. Start slowly, and gradually work harder.

Tummy Shrinker

~ This exercise will help strengthen tummy muscles after your baby comes.

~ Like Kegel exercises, you can do this just about anywhere.

~ Standing or sitting, take a deep breath.

~ While exhaling, tighten tummy muscles as though you were zipping up a pair of tight jeans.

~ Repeat 6 or 8 times.

Orange Crush

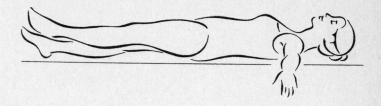

Tones pelvic-floor muscles.

Lie on the floor on your back. Place arms straight out from your sides. Cross one leg over the opposite ankle, and squeeze legs together. Hold 4 seconds, then release. Repeat with legs crossed the opposite way. Do 6 times for each leg.

Torso Twist

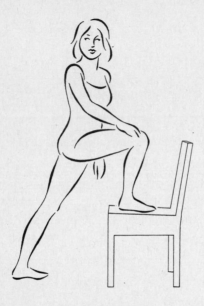

Tones leg and back muscles.

Place a chair in the corner so it won't slide when you push against it. Place right foot on the chair seat; support yourself against the wall with your hand, if necessary. Stretch left leg behind you, lift chest and arch back. Turn shoulders and lean torso to right. Hold 25 to 30 seconds. Do 3 stretches for each side. Do this stretch before beginning tummy exercises.

Tummy Tightener

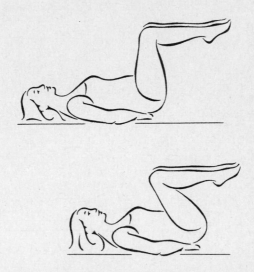

Strengthens tummy muscles.

Lie on your back on the floor. Lift both feet about 18 inches off the floor, bending knees at a right angle. Place hands under hips to support lower back. Raise head slightly, keeping shoulders and upper back on the floor. Bring knees toward face while lifting your feet. Use tummy muscles to lift legs; don't push against the floor with your arms. Hold for a count of 5. Begin by doing 3, and work up to 25.

Lower-Belly Toner

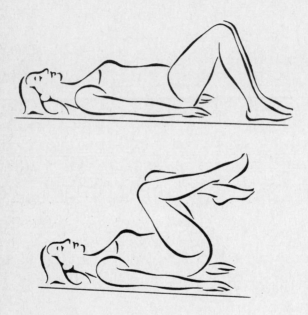

Tones tummy muscles.

Lie on your back on the floor, with hands at sides. Holding feet together, cross ankles, bend knees and lift legs up to a 90° angle. Using tummy muscles, not pushing with your hands, lift hips a few inches off the floor. Hold then release. Work up to 15 repetitions each day.

Closing Flower

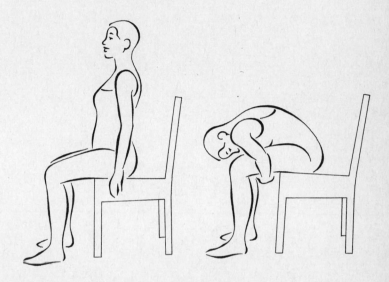

Helps ease tight back muscles.

Sit on the edge of a chair, with knees 6 inches apart and feet facing front. Lean forward until your tummy touches your thighs. Clasp wrists together under your thighs. Breathe deeply through your nose, and let your chin drop onto your chest. Hold for 30 seconds, then push back to upright sitting position. Repeat 3 or 4 times.

Church Steeple

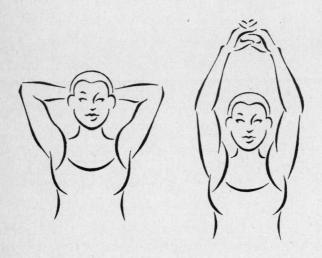

Tones arm and shoulder muscles.

Sit up straight. Lace fingers together behind your head; keep elbows apart. Inhale and push hands, with fingers still together, toward ceiling. Exhale and return hands to position behind your head. Repeat 5 times.

Ballerina Stretch

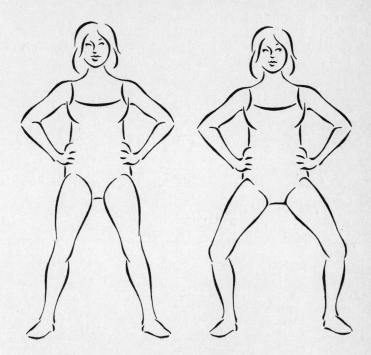

Strengthens and tones leg muscles.

Stand with feet slightly wider than shoulder-width apart. Turn toes out slightly. Place hands on tummy, and slowly squat with knees over toes. Hold for count of 3. Keeping back straight, slowly rise to standing position. Repeat 8 times.

Raise the Bridge

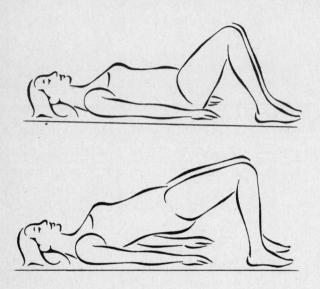

Tones tummy muscles.

Lie on back on the floor, with knees bent and feet flat on the floor. Place hands by your sides, keeping shoulders on floor. Squeezing buttock muscles together, lift hips from floor high enough so that you create a straight line between hips, knees and shoulders. Hold for count of 5, then slowly return hips to floor. Repeat 10 times.

Tummy Crunches

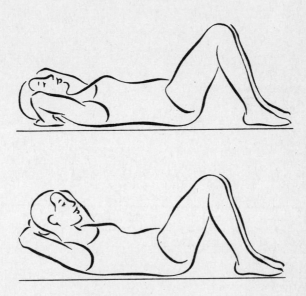

Tones tummy muscles.

Lying on the floor, bend knees and place feet flat on the floor. Place hands under your head. Tighten tummy muscles as you lift head and shoulders slightly. Keep chin open (look forward and up). Hold crunch for 4 seconds. Repeat 10 times.

Side Squeezers

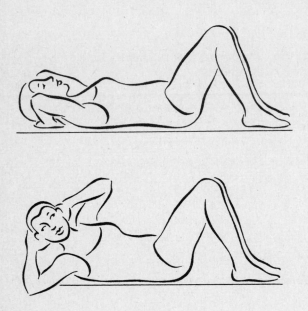

Tightens oblique muscles, which are on the sides of your waist.

To work the sides of your waist, position yourself as for the basic tummy crunch (previous page). When you lift, rotate toward one knee. Hold crunch for 4 seconds, then repeat for other side. Repeat 10 times.

Breast Boosters

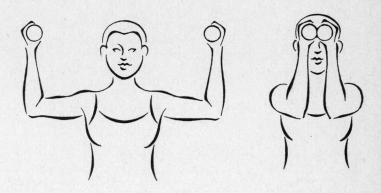

Tightens breast muscles to help keep breasts from sagging.

Sit on the edge of a chair. Using light weights (2 to 3 pounds each to start; if you don't have weights, use a 16-ounce can), raise arms to shoulder level, and bend elbows to point hands toward ceiling. Slowly bring elbows and arms together in front of your face. Hold for 4 seconds, then slowly open to shoulder width. Repeat 8 times; work up to 20 times.

Push Up, Up and Away

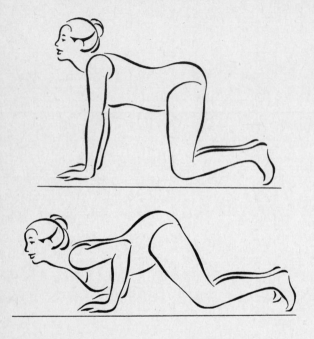

Strengthens arm and back muscles.

Kneel on floor with weight on hands and knees. Bending elbows, lower chest toward floor while inhaling until you are about 2 inches from the floor. Hold for a count of 2. Straighten arms and push back up while exhaling. Hold for a count of 3. Repeat 6 times.

Waist Cincher

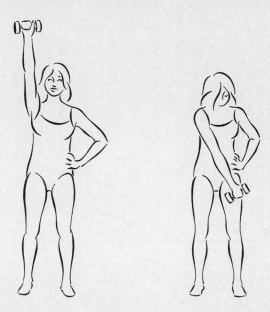

Slims and trims waistline.

Stand with feet apart and knees relaxed. Holding a light weight in your right hand (a 16-ounce can will do fine), extend right arm straight over your head. Contract tummy muscles, bend slightly at the waist then swing arm down and over your left foot. Complete exercise by making a complete circle and returning arm to original position, above your right shoulder. Repeat 8 times on each side.

Chair Can-Can

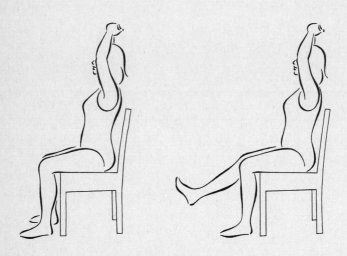

Tones thigh, hip and buttock muscles.

Sit on edge of chair, and place both feet flat on floor.
Relax shoulders, and curve arms over head. Keeping back
straight, hold in tummy muscles while you extend one leg
out in front. Using thigh muscles only, lift leg about 10
inches off the floor. Hold for a count of 5, then slowly
lower foot. Repeat 10 times with each leg.

Bow and Reach

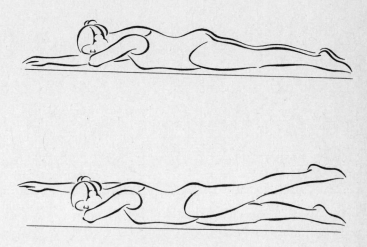

Strengthens back muscles, and tones tummy muscles.

Lie on your tummy with left arm under your forehead. Stretch right hand in front with your palm flat on the floor. Together, slowly lift right hand and left leg off floor. Hold for count of 2, then lower slowly. Repeat 8 times for each side.

Kick Lifts

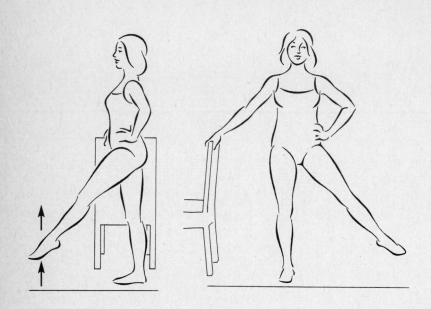

Tones leg and buttock muscles.

Hold onto door jamb or back of a sturdy chair. Beginning with left leg, point your toe and lift leg forward to 90°, then lower to floor. Without stopping, lift same leg to side, as far as you can but not beyond 90°. Return to starting position. Repeat 10 times for each leg.

Buddha Stretch

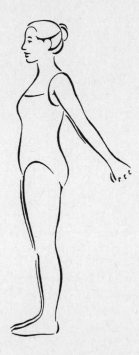

Stretches arm and back muscles, and opens upper chest.

To help improve your posture, stand or sit on the floor, and clasp hands behind you. Lift arms until you feel a good stretch in your upper-chest area and upper arms. Hold for a count of 5, then lower arms. Repeat 8 times.

Elevator Lift

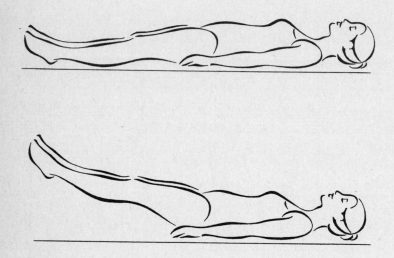

Tones tummy muscles.

Lie on your back on the floor. Keeping both legs together, lift legs slowly from the hip. Be sure you use your tummy muscles for this one. Hold for 6 seconds, then slowly lower both legs to the floor. Work up to 8 repetitions.

Tummy Scrunch

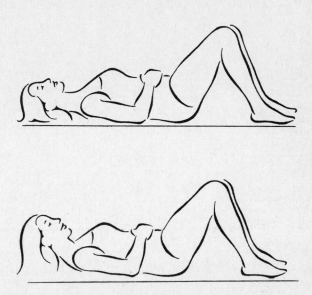

Strengthens tummy muscles.

Lie on your back on the floor, with knees bent and feet flat. Put your hands on your tummy. Suck in your tummy, pulling your navel toward your spine. Hold 4 seconds and release. When you are able to do 8 repetitions, lift your head toward your chest. Hold for 4 seconds, then lower head and hold for 4 seconds. Work up to 10 repetitions.

Bun-and-Back Stretch

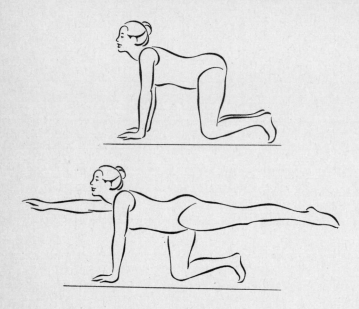

Strengthens buttock, back and leg muscles.

Kneel on hands and knees, with wrists directly beneath shoulders and knees directly beneath hips. Keep your back straight. Contract tummy muscles, then extend left leg behind you at hip height. At same time, extend right arm at shoulder height. Hold 5 seconds, and return to kneeling position. Repeat on other side. Start with 4 repetitions on each side, and gradually work up to 10.

Chair Squat

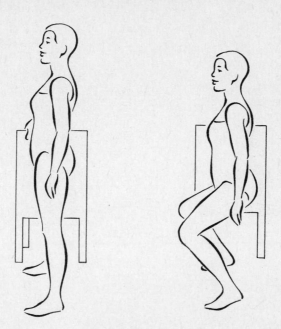

Strengthens hip, thigh and buttock muscles.

Lightly grasp the back of a chair or a counter for balance. Stand with feet shoulder-width apart. Keep torso erect and body weight over heels. Bend knees, and lower torso in squatting position. Don't round your back. Hold squatting position for 5 seconds, then straighten to starting position. Start with 5 repetitions, and work up to 10.

Sit and Dip

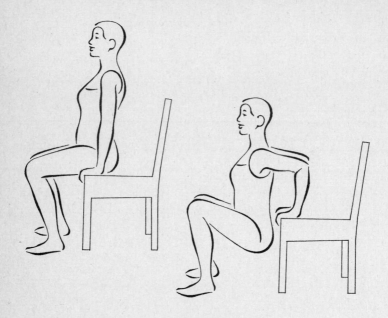

Strengthens and tones arm muscles.

Sit on the edge of a sofa, sturdy chair or sturdy coffee table. Place your hands at your hips, with fingers closed over the edge of the furniture. Walk your feet forward about 1 foot; scoot your bottom off the seat. Bend your elbows to lower your body about 6 inches, keeping your back close to the furniture. Raise up, but don't sit down. Lower yourself again. Begin with 5 repetitions, and increase to 12.

Goal-Post Stretch

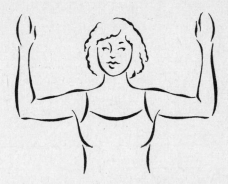

Improves posture, and relieves upper-back stress.

Stand with your feet apart, knees softly bent. Raise arms so upper arms are parallel to the floor and hands point up into the air. Squeeze your shoulder blades together, hold for 3 seconds, then release. Do 10 times.

Baby, the Stroller and Me

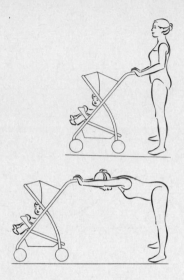

Helps with posture and balance.

Place baby in stroller; place stroller in front of you, with brake off. Stand holding stroller with feet shoulder-width apart and knees soft. Keep your arms close to your body. Straighten arms to push the stroller away slowly. As you push, bend forward from your hips until back is parallel to the floor. Tuck in your tummy, and keep shoulders and head in line with hips. Hold for 5 seconds, then return to standing position by slowly pulling stroller toward you. Repeat 5 times.

Rock the Cradle

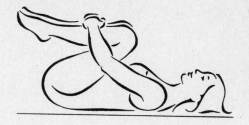

Strengthens and tightens tummy muscles.

Lie on the floor on your back. Bend your knees to your chest, and hold your shins. As you inhale, use hands to pull knees gently toward shoulders. As you exhale, tighten tummy muscles and move knees outward and down (making a circle). Do 10 times.

Baby Bounce

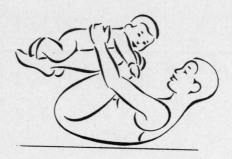

Strengthens and tightens tummy muscles.

Sit on the floor and bend knees, placing feet flat on the floor. Place baby on your lower legs, holding his sides for security. As you tighten tummy muscles, tilt your pelvis and roll backward, lifting feet off the floor and raising baby into the air. In this position, lift head and shoulders off the floor; laugh at baby! Return shoulders and head to the floor, lower baby and legs, and rest. Do 8 times.

Baby Air Lift

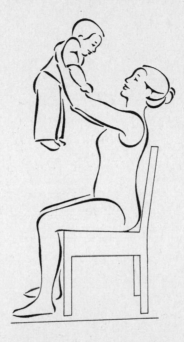

Strengthens shoulder, upper-back and biceps muscles.

Sit on a chair, with knees bent and feet flat on the floor. Hold baby in front of you at chest height. Bend elbows. Tighten tummy muscles for stability, then lift baby while straightening your arms. Gently blow air at him. Return to starting position. Do 10 times.

Baby Hug and Squat

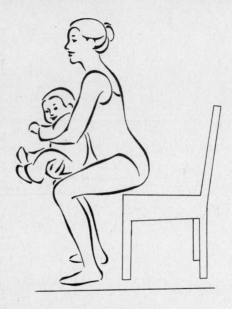

Strengthens leg and buttock muscles.

Holding baby face out and close to your chest, stand with your back to a chair. Tighten tummy muscles, and squeeze shoulders together. Keep back straight and body weight over heels; bend knees and slowly squat toward the chair. You will be leaning forward slightly. When your bottom barely touches the chair seat, slowly return to standing position. Begin with 5 repetitions, and work up to 15.

Relaxation Break

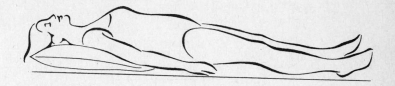

Helps relieve backache, and relaxes you.

Lie on the floor with a pillow placed lengthwise under you. Your head should rest at the top of the pillow. Spread feet shoulder-width apart. Stretch arms and hands out slightly away from your sides. Relax. Let your body go limp, and let your mind wander. Stay in this position for at least 3 minutes.

Also by Glade B. Curtis, M.D., M.P.H., OB/GYN and Judith Schuler, M.S.

Your Pregnancy Week by Week, 5th Edition
ISBN: 1-55561-346-2 (paper)
1-55561-347-0 (cloth)

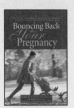

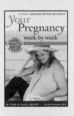

Bouncing Back After Your Pregnancy
ISBN: 0-7382-0606-7

Your Baby's First Year, Week by Week
ISBN: 1-55561-232-6 (paper)
1-55561-257-1 (cloth)

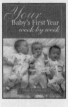

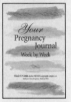

Your Pregnancy Journal Week by Week
ISBN: 1-55561-343-8

Your Pregnancy for the Father to Be
ISBN: 0-7382-1002-1

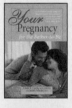

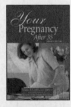

Your Pregnancy After 35
ISBN: 1-55561-319-5

Your Pregnancy Questions and Answers
ISBN: 0-7382-1003-X

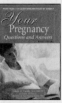

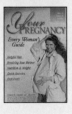

Your Pregnancy: Every Woman's Guide
ISBN: 0-7382-1001-3

Da Capo Lifelong Books are available wherever books are sold and at special discounts for bulk purchases in the U.S. by corporations, institutions, and other organizations. For more information, please contact the Special Markets Department at the Perseus Books Group, 11 Cambridge Center, Cambridge, MA 02142, or call (800) 255-1514, or e-mail special.markets@perseusbooks.com.